I0090417

Clean Eating

Elevate Your Lifestyle Through Nourishing Dietary
Practices For Maximum Physical And Mental Wellness

*(Unveil The Dietary Choices That Enhance And Accelerate
The Tanning Process)*

Columbus Campos

TABLE OF CONTENT

Applying Portion Sizing And Meal Frequency To The Principles Of Clean Eating 1

The Clean Eating Benefits 7

Gaining Comprehension On Weight Reduction And Maintaining Physical Fitness 18

Utilizing Product Labels To Maintain A Healthy Diet 31

Creating A Meal Plan 39

Guidelines On Adopting A Clean Eating Approach In Food Preparation 59

Greek-Style Roast Fish 64

Tips For Getting Started 68

Lemon-Infused Ricotta Dip With Thyme 75

Effective Strategies For Achieving One Month Of Successful Dieting 77

Sweet Potato Waffles..94

Principles Of Clean Eating 97

Balsamic Tomato Bruschetta 106

Creating A Meticulously Crafted Diet Regimen
Tailored To Your Personal Needs, One That
Remains Resiliently Adhered To Over The Span Of
30 Consecutive Days.......................................108

The Significance Of Maintaining Dedication To Your
Dietary Regimen...112

An In-Depth Analysis Of Contemporary Dietary
Patterns...129

Mediterranean Tuna Salad............................148

The Association Between Stress And Weight Gain
....150

Applying Portion Sizing And Meal Frequency To The Principles Of Clean Eating

In addition to consuming nutritious foods, clean eating also emphasizes the cultivation of healthy practices such as appropriate portion control and consistent meal consumption.

Portion Control

Irrespective of the lifestyle or dietary regimen one adheres to, the principle of maintaining appropriate portion sizes consistently emerges. Essentially, portion control encompasses the comprehension of appropriate serving sizes for different types of food. A portion can be measured based on weight, caloric value, or food energy equivalence.

A phenomenon that acts in opposition to the notion of portion control is known as portion distortion. The latter refers to the propensity of individuals to indulge in excess consumption due to the fact that it was provided to them. This matter is highly pervasive within restaurant chains, wherein meals initially designed for an individual consumer are served as platters with the capacity to cater to two or three individuals simultaneously.

Properly regulating serving sizes holds significant significance in all lifestyles, as it effectively mitigates the risk of excessive weight gain and diminishes the likelihood of developing medical conditions associated with this issue.

The difficulty lies in acquiring the knowledge of the appropriate serving size for a specific type of food. This segment poses a challenge, however, there exists a myriad of digital sources and measurement charts that individuals may utilize as valuable tools when embarking on a clean eating journey. When considering portion control, it is imperative that measurements are accurate. Estimates may not be entirely dependable.

Meal Frequency

Omitting meals is not conducive to maintaining good health. Many individuals mistakenly hold the belief that by abstaining from meals, they can regulate their consumption of food and consequently achieve weight loss. This is not a valid assertion. The omission of meals can indeed result in an increase in weight, and the reasons for this are as follows. Upon emerging from a state of repose, such as a restful night's sleep, the body necessitates a surge of vitality in order to initiate proper wakefulness. Consider it akin to inserting a battery into a toy car - without said battery, the car remains motionless.

It is recommended to consume a glass of water and follow it with a sufficient breakfast upon awakening. The term "breakfast" is derived from the expression "to break the fast." The consumption of breakfast initiates the body's metabolic processes, leading to increased calorie burning throughout the day. In the absence of this element, the body will persist in perceiving itself to be in a state of repose.

Furthermore, individuals should refrain from skipping meals due to the subsequent consequences of excessive food intake later in the day. A suitable dietary pattern can be represented by an inverted pyramid, wherein the highest amount of food consumption is recommended during the earlier part of the day, allowing sufficient time for calorie expenditure. When an individual decides to forgo a meal, it disturbs the natural order of their dietary habits, leading to an increased consumption of food during periods nearing their bedtime. Rather than undergoing caloric burn-off, the body opts to store the calories during its resting state, converting them into fat reserves.

In addition to refraining from foregoing meals, it is imperative for individuals to establish a structured meal plan throughout the day. Many individuals have been accustomed to the idea of three main meals per day – breakfast, lunch, and dinner. However, scientific research indicates that consuming five to six small meals throughout the day is more beneficial. Through the adoption of smaller yet frequent meals, there is a consistent dispersion of energy-dense foods at regular intervals. The body receives ample sustenance and efficiently utilizes the energy derived from food, resulting in the absence of excess storage in the form of fat.

The Clean Eating Benefits

More frequently, individuals choose to embrace the clean eating lifestyle driven by their aspiration to shed pounds. Frequently, individuals choose to remain primarily due to the multitude of health advantages that extend beyond mere weight and size reduction.

Recent psychological research indicates that young adults who consume higher quantities of fruits and vegetables exhibit higher levels of "flourishing." This includes increased happiness, positivity, hopefulness, creativity, and a stronger inclination towards personal growth and intellectual curiosity. These identical impacts are subjectively recounted by a multitude of personal trainers and dieticians as they assess the progress of their clients. According to popular belief, irrespective of one's age, practicing a diet that is both nutritious and hygienic has the capacity to cultivate a feeling of wellness, thereby contributing to individuals' strength, concentration, and optimistic outlook.

Additionally, I present to you another set of five profoundly significant advantages associated with adhering to a clean eating regimen. These benefits are entirely independent of one's body size or shape:

1. Improved mood

Additionally, research has been conducted that establishes a correlation between increased consumption of fruits and vegetables and enhanced emotional well-being. Based on the analysis conducted on the dietary patterns and emotional states of a sample size of 300 individuals in the age group of young adults, spanning a duration of 3 weeks, it became evident that an increased consumption of organic foods, specifically fruits and vegetables, led to a notable enhancement in overall emotional well-being, including reduced levels of anxiety, higher energy levels, and increased overall happiness. Additionally, it appeared that the impact of these effects extended beyond the immediate consumption of nutritious food, persisting into the subsequent day.

In recent years, the prevalence of conditions such as depression and anxiety has surged to near-epidemic levels. This alarming trend is evidenced by the staggering statistic that up to 25% of the populace in multiple European nations now rely on anti-depressants or analogous medications to manage their mental well-being. If the promotion of positive emotions is considered a notable advantage of adopting a clean eating regimen, then the widespread adoption of such a lifestyle has the potential to greatly benefit a considerable portion of individuals grappling with mental health issues. Such individuals would be afforded a fresh opportunity to thrive and develop greater resilience to the manifold pressures of contemporary living.

2. Enhanced sleep quality" "Superior sleep experience" "Improved sleep

standards" "Elevated level of sleep" "Enhanced sleep conditions" "Enhanced sleep efficacy" "Optimized sleep experience" "Upgraded sleep standards" "Augmented sleep quality" "Heightened level of sleep

There have been extensive investigations that establish a correlation between a restful night's sleep and enhancements in overall well-being. Additionally, further scientific inquiry indicates that the consumption of appropriate nutrition can contribute significantly to attaining this crucial aspect of sleep quality. For instance, a study conducted in Taiwan revealed that individuals of both genders experiencing sleep-related difficulties could potentially alleviate their symptoms through the consumption of kiwis. Upon the completion of a 4-week duration during which individuals consumed 2 kiwis approximately 1 hour prior to their bedtime, notable improvements in sleep patterns were observed. Specifically, the subjects experienced a 35% decrease in the time it took them to initiate sleep, coupled with a 13% prolongation in their overall sleep duration. Furthermore, individuals reported a profound sense of enhanced sleep quality surpassing any previous experiences.

As anticipated, a multitude of analogous research endeavours have established correlations between numerous nutritious dietary options and enhanced sleep patterns. Included in these dietary options are fish, dark leafy greens, select varieties of nuts, as well as a range of whole grain foods. The predominant notion suggests that enhancing one's dietary habits will likewise enhance their quality of sleep. Enhanced sleep quality directly correlates with an elevated state of well-being.

3. Better workouts

Individuals who prioritize physical fitness are perpetually seeking avenues to enhance their performance during exercise and subsequently maximize their attainable outcomes. Several nutritious and hygienic food options have demonstrated an ability to positively impact muscular growth, expedited recovery periods, and enhanced athletic stamina. A physiological investigation revealed that consistent intake of 16 fluid ounces of organic beetroot juice on a daily basis over a period of 6 days was observed to enhance the cycling performance of athletes. This resulted in an increase in their endurance capacity by up to 16%, which experts assert cannot be solely attributed to physical conditioning efforts. Nutrient-rich foods constitute a significant aspect of the clean eating regimen, and may prove beneficial if you encounter a plateau during your personal fitness routine.

4. Glowing skin

The skin exhibits its appreciation when nourished with pure, wholesome substances. Several studies have indicated that the radiance exhibited by individuals who adhere to a nutritious diet is actually more aesthetically pleasing than the appearance achieved through regular tanning efforts. Additional research has indicated that individuals who consume greater quantities of fruits and vegetables exhibit a heightened level of physical attractiveness compared to those who have a lower intake of such produce. The core idea conveyed is that our physical appearance and internal well-being are greatly influenced by the food we consume. Adhering to a healthy diet will bestow upon you a resplendence that is aesthetically pleasing to observers.

5. Enhanced cognitive abilities

For a considerable duration, it has been widely held that the Mediterranean diet establishes the standard for consuming nutrients in a healthful manner. This diet entails consuming a substantial quantity of fruits and vegetables, in addition to legumes, nuts and seeds, avocado, first-pressed olive oil, and seafood. Include a modest quantity of wine, accompanied by a limited consumption of high-fat meats, dairy items, processed grains, and, significantly, sugar. Research findings indicate that following this dietary regimen has been associated with a decreased incidence of brain infarctions, or localized cerebral tissue necrosis, resulting in potential cognitive impairment mitigation.

Additionally, studies of a similar nature indicate that adhering more closely to the Mediterranean diet can significantly reduce the likelihood of brain damage over an extended period, in contrast to those who adhere least closely to this dietary pattern. Taking a long-term perspective, it reduces the likelihood of developing age-related cognitive impairment, as well as the progression of this impairment to age-related disorders such as dementia and Alzheimer's.

Gaining Comprehension On Weight Reduction And Maintaining Physical Fitness

A significant number of individuals globally are encountering considerable challenges in navigating the issues associated with obesity and excessive weight. The frequency at which these cases are escalating is cause for concern, surpassing any previous temporal records within recent recollection. This matter is of significant magnitude and encompasses various aspects of society and individuals' ways of living. It impacts individuals across all social classes, including both wealthy and impoverished individuals; males and females of all ages. Obesity presents a significant public health concern. When an excessive amount of adipose tissue surpasses the proportion of muscle mass within an individual's body, a plethora of complications tend to manifest.

In the event that an individual is unable to maintain an optimal and balanced weight corresponding to their height, it may greatly augment the risk of developing a range of health conditions, including but not limited to, gallstones, coronary heart diseases, multiple forms of cancer, diabetes, and various other ailments detrimental to one's health.

The fundamental concept of adhering to a clean eating regimen is rooted in the belief that nutritional intake plays a pivotal role in addressing weight loss, surpassing the influence of physical activity and genetic predispositions that are often considered influential factors in shaping our bodies. The consumption of wholesome food inherently brings forth discernible outcomes that manifest themselves on both physiological and aesthetic levels.

I do not intend to imply that there may be individuals who advocate for the recommendation of supplements or other medications deemed effective. Nevertheless, it is feasible to achieve weight loss through natural means. Ultimately, it pertains to the employment of sanitary practices.

Please find below two techniques that will enable you to determine if your weight is appropriate for your height, as well as whether your body weight and fat level are conducive to maintaining a state of overall health and well-being.

Assessing Body Fat: The standard range for Body Mass Index (BMI) that indicates average or healthy levels falls within the range of 18.5-25. When an individual's BMI exceeds 25, it is classified as being overweight, and if it surpasses 30, it is recognized as obesity.

You can effortlessly calculate your BMI by employing this uncomplicated mathematical equation:

There are several varied methods available to determine your body's percentage of adipose tissue: you may opt to measure the water displacement caused by submerging yourself in a hydrostatic tank, or you can utilize a device resembling a bathroom scale specifically designed for this purpose. Additional fundamental techniques for accomplishing this at one's residence entail the utilization of 'Bio electrical Impedance' or the 'Waist-to-hip ratio'.

Assessing your Waist-to-Hip Ratio: Observing the presence of adipose tissue distributed throughout the body can serve as a reliable indicator of obesity or overweight conditions. An ample amount of adipose tissue tends to accumulate in the abdominal region of individuals with obesity, and this can give rise to potential health hazards such as an increased susceptibility to weight-related illnesses.

In order to conduct the calculation, it is necessary to measure (in inches or cm) the circumference of your waist at its narrowest point that can be readily identified just above your navel. Please record the estimated measurement, and subsequently perform the same action around the broadest region of your hips.

The waist to hip ratio is determined by dividing the waist measurement by the hip measurement.

A health alert is indicated for individuals of average constitution when the proportion exceeds 0.94. For an average woman, a ratio of 0.82 or higher indicates a state of peril.

Kindly be advised that, for the sake of utmost accuracy, it is recommended that you obtain three distinct assessments for each aforementioned component. When performing calculations, it is recommended to utilize the smallest of the three estimates obtained from your waist and pair it with the largest estimate obtained from your waist.

The Significance of Weight Reduction and Maintaining Physical Fitness

Enhances vitality: This transformation in your physical well-being is readily discernible. By engaging in a variety of physical activities and adhering to a nutritious dietary regime, you will gradually experience a noticeable enhancement in your overall vitality. Throughout the entirety of the day, you will experience both a heightened sense of alertness and revitalization. If one adopts a lifestyle that is characterized by a lack of physical activity and a general state of inactivity, it will result in feelings of fatigue and lethargy throughout the entirety of the day.

Enhancement of Digestive System: Incorporating physical activities and adopting healthy dietary practices significantly contribute to the optimization of the digestive process, thereby mitigating the occurrence of obstructions and various digestive disorders. The elimination of excess fats and the incorporation of low-fat nutrition serves as a preventive measure against ailments such as diabetes, hypertension, and other associated disorders.

General well-being is significantly improved by adhering to a regular fitness regimen and adopting a nutritious dietary plan. The beneficial impacts will gradually manifest once you establish a consistent training routine and consume nutritionally balanced meals. Engaging in a regular routine of brisk walking for a duration of 30 minutes is adequately effective in maintaining your physical fitness. Engaging in physical training enhances blood circulation within the body and fortifies the immune system.

Enhances Physical Strength: Engaging in regular exercise routines and following balanced dietary practices not only promote overall fitness, but also contribute to the growth of muscles and the fortification of bones. Individuals who encounter the adverse effects of shoulder pain, spinal discomfort, and similar ailments should engage in regular and substantial physical activity. If you maintain regularity in your physical activities, the intensity of the discomfort will assuredly diminish. You will understand the importance of physical fitness in improving muscular strength.

Enhances psychological resilience: Physical fitness encompasses not only physical attributes but also cultivates mental fortitude. Incorporating a combination of general physical activity and adopting a well-balanced dietary approach will enhance cognitive function through the facilitation of cerebral blood circulation. It enhances cerebral blood flow, thereby improving cognitive function and memory. In order to fully reap the benefits, one must engage in consistent practice.

Improving physical fitness: This represents a notable benefit of engaging in weight loss and adopting nutritious dietary patterns. Maintaining regular engagement in physical exercises and adhering to a balanced nutritional regimen are widely considered as the most effective and prevalent approaches for achieving weight loss. You will effectively burn calories and decrease caloric consumption, thereby promoting a beneficial state of health for your body. You will also maintain optimum physical health.

Cardiovascular health: This refers to the assessment of the heart's vitality at its core. Similarly, it also implies the body's ability to transport additional nutrients and oxygen to the bloodstream's tissues, while simultaneously eliminating waste from the body. Engaging in regular exercise and maintaining a nutritious diet enable the attainment of cardiovascular fitness, while also fostering a consistent supply of oxygen to all the body's muscles.

Enhances your self-assurance and self-worth: Maintaining physical fitness contributes to cultivating a positive perception of oneself. The greater your persistent efforts towards achieving a healthy lifestyle, the more you enhance your overall physical appearance. This will enhance your sense of identity and elevate your level of confidence. Throughout the entire day, you will experience rejuvenation and an invigorating sensation. Furthermore, you shall maintain an optimistic outlook and experience an abundance of joy.

Utilizing Product Labels To Maintain A Healthy Diet

We have established that adhering to a clean diet is an effective method of detoxifying one's body. However, it is possible to contend that maintaining a healthy diet is a costly endeavor for some individuals. Allow me to present a highly significant element in this context. Although organic products do come with a higher price tag compared to their non-organic counterparts, it is important to note a significant caveat. When purchasing items such as tomatoes and tuna, for instance, selecting those that have been cultivated without the use of antibiotics, hormones, synthetic nutrients, and similar substances. You would be remunerating an equal amount for both a canned meat with spaghetti sauce, enhanced by the addition of maltodextrin. However, the former option is capable of imbuing you with a greater level of vigor, unlike the latter that elicits increased hunger and diminished energy. Therefore, products that are not organic, refined, or subjected to chemical processing are unable to fulfill the primary purpose of food, namely, providing us with the necessary energy. Consequently, you expend money on sustenance that fails to satiate your hunger and merely engenders a desire for additional consumption, thereby entailing a twofold payment for a larger quantity of food. Is that the objective of your visit to the supermarket? If you find yourself lacking interest in this notion, it would be advantageous for you to commence reading the labels in order to safeguard yourself against the deceptive practices of the manufacturer.

The primary guideline when perusing the labels entails having the capacity to comprehend and articulate the constituents. If the tomato sauce packaging specifies the presence of tomato, garlic, basil, and olive oil – all ingredients with easily discernible names that you would willingly purchase individually from a store to prepare the same sauce at your own domicile, it can be deemed a consummate manifestation of cleanliness. However, should the ingredient list contain substances such as Ractopamine, Monosodium Glutamate (MSG), Aspartame, or any other components not inherently produced by nature, it is recommended to abstain from consuming said product. Ultimately, would you be inclined to visit the store with the intention of purchasing Ractopamine?

Please bear in mind that the quality of blueberries surpasses that of blueberry syrup, fresh garlic is preferable over garlic powder, whole apples are superior to apple mixes, and tomatoes are more desirable than tomato extract or concentrate, among other examples.

Beware the following chemicals:

Artificial sweeteners, namely Aspartame, Splenda, Acesulfame Potassium, Neotame, and Saccarin

Artificial color additives, including Brilliant Blue, Fast Green, Indigotine, Erythrosine, Tartrazine, Sunset Yellow, and Allura Red.

Artificial flavors encompass a range of aromatic, heteroaromatic, and heterocyclic chemical compounds that are not obtained from natural sources such as spices, fruits, herbs, buds, leaves, barks, roots, or edible yeast, in other words, substances derived solely from Nature.

Trans fatty acids, such as Hydrogenated or partially hydrogenated vegetable oils, glyphosate.

Preservation agents, encompassing antimicrobial substances, antioxidants, and chelating agents like sulphites, sorbates, benzoates, and nitrates, as well as TBHQ (tertiary-butyl hydroquinone), BHA, and BHT (butylated hydroxyanisole and hydroxytoluene).

Ingredients that have been genetically modified or genetically engineered, typically abbreviated as GE, should not be subject to engineering processes, but rather should be cultivated.

Monosodium Glutamate (MSG), along with any substances that have been hydrolyzed, enzyme modified or fermented, protein concentrates, isolates or extracts, as well as Vestin, Gelatin, Umami and all additives with the letter "E".

Please ensure to monitor the expiration date of the product. If the expiration date on the sour-cream label indicates a period of two weeks (which is rather unusual), and the product is nearing the aforementioned duration yet maintains its visual quality, it can be inferred that the sour cream has been artificially preserved.

Lastly, it is advantageous to procure your fruits and vegetables from local farmers' markets rather than from conventional supermarkets. Enormous strawberries, impeccably uniform mushrooms, and lustrous oranges on the brink of rupture are inherently inferior to their organic, typical-sized equivalents.

So let's sum up. No abbreviations will be found within the ingredients list, as they are likely to consist of chemical substances. Our products do not contain any artificial additives, and our fruits are not unnaturally oversized or artificially enhanced to appear glossy. Furthermore, our products are free from any additives marked with the symbol 'E', and their expiry dates are not excessively extended. Pretty simple, isn't it?

Creating A Meal Plan

If you have consistently maintained an unhealthy diet, you may encounter considerable challenges when attempting to adopt a nutritious eating regimen. Nonetheless, there is no need for concern, as with unwavering determination and steadfast discipline, you can indeed triumph in this undertaking.

Consuming nutritious food does not require excessive sophistication. It is imperative to acquire high-quality ingredients, namely grass-fed beef and organic produce. If you find yourself having a particularly busy schedule, it would be advisable to engage in grocery shopping at least three days in advance, thereby allowing ample time for food preparation and cooking without unnecessary haste.

Please refrain from being overly concerned with the excessive preparation of food. One can invariably preserve the remaining portions for future use or opt to distribute them among relatives and acquaintances. However, there is no necessity for you to meticulously assess the weight and proportions of your meals. Please indulge in as much food as you desire, on the condition that your choices align with a nutritious and balanced diet. Please ensure the incorporation of nutritious fats, carbohydrates, and proteins in combination.

Useful Advice for Developing a Dietary Schedule

An effective guideline to adhere to when planning your meals is to ensure that forty percent of your carbohydrate intake is derived from fruits and vegetables, while allocating thirty percent to lean sources of protein and the remaining thirty percent to dietary fat. It is imperative to exercise caution while consuming fruits, particularly if your aim is weight loss. While fruits boast nutritional value, they also tend to exhibit elevated levels of sugar.

It is advisable to exercise moderation when consuming certain fruits such as mangoes, bananas, grapes, and oranges. These fruits possess significant levels of fructose, which undergo direct hepatic metabolism akin to that of alcohol. It would be advisable to exercise moderation when consuming dried fruits, including raisins, as they contain significant levels of sugars. However, it is permissible to consume cherries, apples, and berries in unlimited quantities. Blueberries, strawberries and raspberries are highly suitable choices for nourishing snacks and delectable desserts. They possess a rich assortment of phytonutrients and dietary fiber.

Despite financial constraints, it is still possible to maintain a nutritious diet. Insufficient financial resources should not impede one's ability to attain good health. One can optimize their financial resources by purchasing meat, eggs, and seafood. These food items occupy the highest position in the food hierarchy.

Go for colorful produce. The consumption of a diverse assortment of vegetables and fruits offers multiple health benefits for the human body. Not only do their vibrant hues enhance their visual appeal, but they also serve as an indication that these fruits and vegetables are rich in essential nutrients. An example would be the abundance of beta carotene found in sweet potatoes, as opposed to the substantial lycopene content found in tomatoes.

Do not be deceived by food items that portray themselves as whole grains. When perusing the assortment of snack bars and crackers at the supermarket, it is not uncommon to encounter the terms 'fiber' and 'wheat' listed among the ingredients delineated on their respective labels. These food products may not possess inherent nutritional qualities, despite their assertions of being healthy. For individuals seeking a nutritious breakfast or snack, it is advisable to opt for unprocessed whole grains such as quinoa, whole wheat flour, and rolled or steel cut oats.

Additionally, it is advisable to examine the roster of constituents in order to ascertain whether or not they consist of whole foods, rather than synthetic and extensively refined ingredients. It is crucial to refrain from consuming artificial food coloring, artificial sweeteners, and partially hydrogenated oil, particularly in your diet. It is imperative that you refrain from consuming foods that are enriched with excessive amounts of salt, fat, and sugar.

In addition, it is crucial to integrate lean proteins into one's diet. Health-conscious individuals often opt for lean ground beef and chicken breast, however, it is advisable to consider diversifying your culinary repertoire without hesitation. Permissible options for consumption include tilapia, wild salmon, catfish, as well as a variety of seeds and nuts. Refrain from consuming cold cuts containing elevated levels of nitrates and sodium.

It is recommended to utilize either organic expeller-pressed canola oil or extra virgin olive oil for your cooking oil. Additionally, expeller-pressed peanut oil, avocado oil, and grape seed oil are viable alternatives. If you have a preference for utilizing butter in your culinary endeavors, then virgin coconut oil can be a highly suitable substitute. However, it is advised to exercise moderation when incorporating it into your recipes.

Whenever feasible, opt for meat products that are antibiotic-free. This implies that it is imperative for you to purchase meat that originates from pigs or chickens that have not been subjected to antibiotic treatment. Excessive usage of antibiotics in animals has the potential to diminish their efficacy in humans. To ensure consumption of healthy meats, it is advisable to opt for organic alternatives.

There is no necessity for you to entirely eradicate fats from your dietary intake. One must simply opt for nutritious fats in lieu of saturated fats. Canola oil, olive oil, fatty fish, and nuts are sources of nutritious fats, whereas butter and cheese contain saturated fats. Nutritious fats are, in fact, beneficial for cardiovascular health and demonstrate efficacy in promoting elevated levels of beneficial HDL cholesterol. Conversely, saturated fats have been found to be associated with cardiovascular diseases.

What methods can be utilized to determine the presence of saturated fats? Easy. In the event that the fats undergo a transformation into a solid state when exposed to room temperature, they can be classified as saturated fats. You can reduce your consumption of these unhealthy fats by replacing certain food items in your dietary regimen. As an example, rather than incorporating cheese into your salad, you have the option to add nuts instead. In lieu of cream cheese, peanut butter can serve as a suitable alternative; similarly, avocado can be substituted for mayonnaise in your sandwich.

Maintaining a wholesome dietary regimen necessitates minimizing alcohol consumption as well. If it is not feasible to entirely eradicate it from your dietary habits, please restrict your consumption to a maximum of two beverages daily for men and one beverage per day for women. Please take note that a volume of five ounces of wine is equal to a single alcoholic beverage. In a comparable manner, a single drink is constituted by twelve ounces of beer.

Consuming alcohol in moderation, particularly red wine, can potentially have beneficial effects on cardiovascular health. Excessive consumption can lead to dehydration and contribute to calorie intake. Beverages that possess an excessive amount of sugar pose a particular hazard to one's well-being.

With regards to excessive sugar consumption, it is recommended by the

American Heart Association to restrict one's daily sugar intake to nine teaspoons for men and six teaspoons for women. Control your consumption of confectioneries, pastries, and carbonated beverages, while opting for healthier alternatives such as unsweetened yogurt in lieu of ice cream.

Similar to sugar, excessive consumption of salt can pose health risks. It is observed that the sodium consumption of Americans often exceeds the threshold of two thousand and three hundred milligrams on a daily basis, consequently rendering them particularly prone to suffering from hypertension. Decrease your sodium intake by restricting your consumption of processed and packaged foods. If one desires to enhance the taste of their culinary preparations, they may opt for the utilization of herbs, spices, vinegar, and citrus alongside, as opposed to relying solely on the inclusion of salt.

Consuming a diet that prioritizes clean and nutritious foods offers numerous advantages for one's overall well-being. This is the underlying cause that motivates a multitude of individuals to endeavor this dietary approach. It constitutes an essential element of maintaining a wholesome way of life. Presented below are several discernible advantages associated with the practice of consuming clean and unprocessed foods.

Improve Health and Wellbeing

Consuming food that is free from artificial or chemical additives, and instead consists of all-natural ingredients, contributes to the enhancement of one's well-being as it aids in maintaining good health. Processed food toxins are responsible for a myriad of illnesses, including but not limited to cancer, cardiovascular conditions, and diabetes. Clean eating further supports the cultivation of a well-rounded diet by advocating for the consumption of appropriate quantities of essential nutrients. If one ensures that the body receives adequate nourishment, its immune system will be fortified, thus safeguarding it against various ailments. Furthermore, by opting for a reduced meat consumption and selectively choosing high-quality meat, you will also experience a notable decrease in the pressure on your physique, resulting in a lighter bodily sensation. Certain individuals choose to abstain from consuming meat altogether, opting to obtain their protein needs from alternative sources. However, the determination to make such a decision ultimately lies in your own hands. Furthermore, abstaining from meat consumption can serve as a preventive measure against health conditions resulting from excessive meat intake, such as hypertension and cardiovascular accidents.

In addition to enhancing your physical well-being, adhering to a clean dietary regimen also contributes to the improvement of your mental well-being. This can be attributed to the fact that you are receiving essential nutrients that are crucial for your bodily requirements, thereby significantly enhancing your overall mood and emotional state. In addition, it aids in the mitigation of depressive symptoms and the alleviation of anxiety.

Lose Weight

The adherence to clean eating practices facilitates weight loss as it entails consuming appropriate quantities of fulfilling, nutrient-rich food. This holds particularly true when consuming minimal quantities of meat as it has the potential to contribute to an increase in body weight. There is no requirement for you to attempt those exorbitant dietary trends that gain popularity annually. Minimal effort is required when adopting a clean eating approach. Individuals who do not actively pursue weight loss are able to effortlessly shed excess fat and attain their ideal weight through adhering to the tenets of clean eating. Clean eating also promotes the consumption of five to six smaller meals throughout the day, as opposed to three larger meals. This approach promotes a lasting sense of satiety and contentment throughout the day, consequently discouraging the indulgence in snacks and sweets as a means to fulfill cravings and alleviate hunger.

Boost Energy

In present times, individuals often experience heightened fatigue due to their predominantly inactive way of life. You frequently experience a post-prandial decline. This can similarly be ascribed to your poor dietary habits. If the majority of your diet primarily comprises refined sugar, you will experience notable fluctuations in energy levels that tend to diminish in the afternoon, resulting in feelings of lethargy following lunch. By adopting a dietary modification and embracing a regimen of consuming nutritious foods, you will experience a surge in energy levels, subsequently enhancing your productivity. Furthermore, if one possesses a heightened sense of vigor, there is a greater likelihood of engaging in physical activity, thus facilitating the enhancement of energy levels, the reduction of weight, and the attainment of optimal well-being.

Guidelines On Adopting A Clean Eating Approach In Food Preparation

The pursuit of maintaining a healthy diet can occasionally prove disheartening, even for individuals already well-versed in culinary practices. For individuals who are beginners in the culinary world, these suggestions are undoubtedly capable of amplifying your enthusiasm to create healthier renditions of your preferred dishes as well as exploring novel recipes.

Enhance Your Meals: If you feel a sense of apprehension towards experimenting with various spices and seasoning combinations, why not consider incorporating herbs and other ingredients that can heighten and transform your nutritious dishes significantly? Consider undertaking culinary trials, by integrating these nutritious herbs and spices into your upcoming gastronomic endeavors:

Cloves

Cinnamon

Nutmeg

Cumin

Turmeric

Sage

Mint

Rosemary

Basil

Marjoram

Chili

Thyme

Devise a meal plan – there are numerous approaches to adding variety to your daily meals. Utilize the internet as a valuable resource, or consult this book, in order to discover delectable and wholesome recipes that can be effortlessly prepared for your loved ones. One can devise a chart and strategize their culinary preparations and dietary choices for a span of seven days or the forthcoming days.

Engage in culinary exploration – embrace venturing beyond your culinary comfort zone and explore a variety of nutritious recipes that you have come across. It is suggested that you initially sample modest servings and evaluate whether both you and the entire household find the dish agreeable.

Prepare your meals in advance – there is no need to subject yourself to daily kitchen obligations, as there exist options for nutritious meals that can be prepared ahead, stored in the refrigerator, and reheated when needed. One can also affix labels on the containers indicating the specific dates or designated days for consumption in order to preserve their freshness and preserve their original flavors.

Create a comprehensive inventory while refraining from excessive enthusiasm regarding the selection of fruits, vegetables, meats, and dairy items. Maintain a comprehensive inventory of your ingredients, ensuring to diligently observe their respective expiration dates. This compiled record will serve as an invaluable point of reference for your next grocery shopping excursion.

Considering all these factors, it is undoubtedly the appropriate moment to commence the culinary process.

Greek-Style Roast Fish

Ingredients:

1 fresh onion

½ fresh lemon

½ teaspoon dried oregano

A handful of parsley

5 potatoes

2 tomatoes

2 skinless Pollock fillets

2 tablespoons of olive oil

2 garlic cloves

Directions:

The potatoes, tomatoes, and fresh lemons should be sliced into wedges. Cut the fresh onion into thin slices and finely dice the garlic and parsley. Preheat the oven to a temperature of 200°C, then proceed to place the olive oil, potatoes, garlic, fresh onion, and oregano inside the roasting tin. Incorporate an assortment of seasonings and combine them diligently with your hands to ensure a comprehensive coating. Subject the dish to a duration of fifteen minutes of roasting, followed by turning it over and baking for an additional fifteen minutes. Incorporate the tomatoes and fresh lemons, then proceed to roast the ingredients for a duration of ten minutes. In conclusion, place the fish fillets on top and proceed to cook for an additional duration of ten minutes. Garnish with finely diced parsley and savor the dish.

Tips For Getting Started

If you are new to the concept of clean eating, it is advisable to acquaint yourself with valuable insights that will facilitate your initial journey. These recommendations will facilitate the transition from your previous dietary patterns and eating habits to the practice of clean eating with greater ease.

Elucidate Your Definition of Clean Eating

As previously delineated in earlier sections, the notion of clean eating exhibits a degree of subjectivity as it diverges across individuals. It is imperative to establish your own distinctive interpretation that will function as a compass when purchasing sustenance and preparing culinary delicacies. The principles of clean eating serve as a fundamental framework, which can be customized to align more effectively with individualized requirements and preferences. A notable illustration would be the adherence to a fundamental tenet of clean eating, which involves the consumption of abundant quantities of fruits and vegetables. Should you desire to incorporate meat into your diet, it is permissible to do so, as the principles of clean eating do not categorically prohibit its consumption. Ensure that you consume lean meat of superior quality.

Ensure your Pantry is well-supplied with Nutritious Food Options

Given that you are embarking on this novel dietary approach, it would be advisable to address the contents of your pantry and refrigerator. It is highly probable that they currently contain a plethora of processed edibles replete with artificial additives. Deplete your pantry and refrigerator of consumables containing artificial components and evident indications of factory processing. One could verify the label and examine the ingredients for this item.

After completing the task of organizing your pantry and fridge, it is advised that you proceed with the activity of purchasing groceries. Certain individuals may encounter difficulty when composing a grocery list comprised solely of items that facilitate clean eating. However, the process can be fundamentally straightforward. Incorporate an abundant assortment of freshly harvested fruits and vegetables, and opt for food items that possess the term 'whole' within their labeling, such as whole wheat bread, whole wheat crackers, or whole grain pasta. An additional term to be mindful of is 'unsweetened', denoting products like almond milk, coconut milk, soy milk, and the like, which lack added sweeteners.

When encountering food items that may be challenging to locate, such as commercially clean ketchup, it is advisable to contemplate the preparation of homemade ketchup utilizing pristine tomatoes and other untainted constituents. It is crucial to adequately prepare for the shopping excursion, particularly if it is your inaugural experience, by methodically composing a grocery list and conducting preliminary investigations on food products amenable to self-preparation.

Allow yourself sufficient time to acclimate.

Shifting from a lifestyle characterized by unrestricted dietary choices to a more regimented approach like adhering to clean eating can pose challenges for individuals, particularly as they come to appreciate the level of effort associated with carefully selecting suitable foods and consistently preparing their own meals. However, as you adapt to this practice and begin to experience the positive outcomes associated with consuming wholesome foods, you will find that everything becomes markedly more effortless. Kindly ensure that you allocate ample time for yourself to adapt. As an illustration, it is not mandatory to completely abandon all your preferred packaged edibles abruptly, such as pizza, cake, or doughnuts. You may continue to consume these foods during your ongoing transition towards adopting a clean eating regimen. As you gradually acclimate to your newfound dietary regimen, you may consider gradually eliminating these processed foods from your consumption repertoire. You can access pristine recipes for your preferred dishes, enabling you to prepare them in the comfort of your own home, utilizing healthy and wholesome ingredients.

If you are contemplating initiating a clean eating lifestyle, it is essential to acquaint yourself with the following information. The following chapter comprises a selection of readily executable recipes suitable for family meals, even amidst a busy schedule.

Lemon-Infused Ricotta Dip With Thyme

Ingredients:

2 teaspoons of fresh lemon zest

¼ cup of freshly squeezed fresh lemon juice

½ teaspoon of sea salt

1 teaspoon of black or white pepper

2 teaspoons of extra virgin olive oil

1 15 ounce container of fresh, part skim ricotta cheese

2 tablespoons of fresh thyme chopped

2 tablespoons of shallot, minced or chopped finely

1 teaspoon of fresh chives, chopped

Instructions

Using either a blender, food processor, or a standard mixer, combine the ricotta cheese, thyme, chives, shallots, fresh lemon zest and juice, salt, and pepper. Whip the ingredients together until they achieve a light and smooth consistency.

Transfer to a bowl and gently garnish with 2 teaspoons of olive oil. Accompany with a side of fresh vegetables, wheat thins, naan bread, or tortilla chips.

Effective Strategies For Achieving One Month Of Successful Dieting

Promoting Nourishing Practices for Optimal Nutrition

Habit 1

Consume six evening meals per day, spaced at an interval of one every two hours. I am aware that the concept may appear remarkable and contrary to the commonly advocated principles of renowned diets, yet consuming nutritious foods with greater frequency in fact enhances your metabolism and sustains elevated levels of energy throughout the entire day. Consuming small meals throughout the day will also stabilize blood sugar levels and curb cravings. Consuming fewer than three meals a day can result in a sudden decrease in your blood sugar levels, rendering you more susceptible to indulging in unhealthy snack choices.

I prefer to compare the digestive system with a smoldering flame of wood. As you persist in adding more wood to the fire, what direction will the flame take? Indeed, veracity surpasses imagination, persist in your resolute pursuit. In the event that you cease adding wood to the fire, what will transpire? The fact has been revealed and it will be disseminated. This bears close resemblance to the digestive system. If you strive to abstain from food with the aim of losing weight, your metabolism will experience a significant decline or deceleration. Once you consume food during that particular moment, your body will proceed to store and retain every ounce in a desperate effort to preserve its well-being. Therefore, it is advisable to meticulously maintain your digestive system in order to ensure its optimal functionality.

Adopting Healthful Practices for Nourishing Nutrition

Habit 2

It is essential to always attend meals, especially the morning meal. What percentages of individuals in your demographic choose to forego breakfast? The examination reveals that individuals who choose to forgo breakfast tend to experience weight gain. Although you may believe that you are economizing on calories, abstaining from breakfast can result in snacking prior to lunch or overindulging during lunch due to your hunger.

Habit 3

Make an effort to refrain from consuming nutritionally empty, high-calorie foods. Processed and fast foods, such as French fries, potato chips, pastries, biscuits, and sweets, represent a nutritional void. The caloric content of these foods is considered "devoid" as they provide a rapid energy boost but lack essential vitamins, nutrients, or natural ingredients. Typically, one tends to experience a surge in energy followed by a subsequent depletion, leading to a diminished state of vitality and increased hunger shortly thereafter. These food items incline towards inducing cravings for considerably higher amounts of energy due to the lack of feeling satiated.

Embarking on the pursuit of a minimalist lifestyle

In contrast to adopting various other dietary approaches, the process of transitioning to a lean lifestyle can be comparatively seamless, contingent upon the level of dedication one already possesses when it comes to consuming predominantly wholesome, unprocessed foods. Nevertheless, if you have a strong inclination towards processed foods, it is regrettable to inform you that the upcoming weeks may pose certain challenges. Many processed foods nowadays contain excessively high amounts of fat and sugar, making a substantial number of them inherently addictive.

This implies that upon making a firm decision to thoroughly purge your refrigerator and completely replace unhealthy options with nutritious alternatives, you will experience the physiological manifestations of withdrawal, akin to individuals undergoing the detoxification process from detrimental substances like drugs or alcohol. Therefore, you have the option to anticipate an unpleasant period of approximately one week during which your body may exhibit flu-like symptoms, or alternatively, gradually eliminate the less healthy components of your diet to minimize discomfort and facilitate a smoother transition.

If one chooses to gradually reduce their dependence, it is critical to abstain from adopting a partially committed approach to adhering to the lean diet, but rather to persevere until achieving a healthier level of sugar and fat intake prior to fully embracing the new dietary regimen. It is not advisable to commence the lean diet in a partial manner as it necessitates wholehearted commitment to specific protein and healthy fat levels, which cannot be ensured if processed foods are still included in the regimen. Do not provide yourself with an escape route when it comes to abandoning your newly adopted lifestyle prematurely, instead exert maximum effort when circumstances allow for it.

Once you are prepared to commence, it is crucial to ensure your future self's convenience and capture a series of preliminary photographs and measurements. This will assist you in your long-term commitment by providing a chance to reflect on your progress and how much you have achieved. Consequently, it is necessary to utilize a weighing scale to assess one's weight in conjunction with evaluating their present muscle mass and body fat. Don't forget to measure your shoulders, chest, waist, calves, thighs and arms for the best results.

Although it might initially pose a challenge to introspect in a highly analytical manner, rest assured that in a few weeks, you will appreciate the value of having a reference point against which to gauge your progress. Please record your present measurements and place them in a location that you will regularly observe upon awakening each day. Subsequently, document the updated measurements each time they are taken, maintaining consistent placement of the record. This graphical depiction of the chronological sequence will greatly facilitate the process of transitioning to the new way of life with a higher likelihood of achieving success.

Adhering to a frugal way of living.

After implementing the prescribed framework outlined within this book, it will be imperative for you to exert deliberate effort in order to establish fresh objectives if you aspire to sustain the lean lifestyle over an extended duration. When selecting objectives, it is crucial to opt for those that are attainable in order to prevent oneself from experiencing discouragement or disillusionment. This implies a reduction in weight ranging from 1 to 1.5 pounds. over the course of each week in the long run, concurrently with the development of muscle mass. Anything beyond that not only lacks feasibility, but also presents a significant threat.

Rather than fixating on exact measurements on the scale, direct your attention towards increasing the number of repetitions or sets during your workout sessions, or observing how a particular garment fits you at different stages of your progress. It is crucial to consistently rely on external influences that steer you towards adopting the mindset required to sustain regular exercise and transform it into a lifelong habit.

Likewise, it is important to be realistic about the fact that, now and then, you won't have the impregnable willpower required to stop yourself from eating something so delicious and so bad for you. In the event that the aforementioned healthy alternatives fail to divert your attention from a particular temptation, it would be advisable to instead focus on minimizing the negative impact to the greatest extent achievable. Please obtain only one cupcake instead of 20.

As long as you exercise moderation, there is no justification for experiencing any guilt regarding your indulgence. Instead, reflect upon the significant improvement in your overall well-being in comparison to when you embarked on this journey. In these instances of indulgence, it is crucial to not allow the deviation from established practices to become the catalyst for regressing into unfavorable conduct. Indulging occasionally is acceptable, provided that you possess the restraint to ensure it remains infrequent.

Consider Carb Cycling

If you wish to enhance the weight loss capabilities of your newly embraced lean lifestyle, you may contemplate incorporating carb cycling as an additional strategy. Carbohydrate cycling involves implementing a distinct dietary approach characterized by the alternating intake of carbohydrates on specific days. Similar to the minimalist approach to dieting, carb cycling centers around consuming nutritious and unprocessed foods and adhering to a regimen of three substantial meals along with two supplementary snacks that are high in protein. Furthermore, it encourages the process of natural weight reduction and the development of lean muscle, all the while enhancing your metabolism – traits that align with the principles of a healthy and slender way of living.

The practice of carb cycling entails strategically consuming higher amounts of carbohydrates on specific days, thus ensuring the replenishment of necessary fuel reserves to sustain energy levels during subsequent low carbohydrate days. Over a period of time, this establishes a situation in which your body initiates the combustion of a greater quantity of calories on the days with higher carbohydrate intake, and gradually adapts to burning that elevated calorie amount on the days with lower carbohydrate intake, which eventually manifest with increased frequency.

To initiate carb cycling, one may commence by alternating between days of greater carbohydrate consumption and days of lesser carbohydrate intake. Moreover, during the days of increased carbohydrate consumption, it is permissible to indulge in a single item of one's choice, provided it is not consumed during the evening hours. Commencing from Monday, incorporate a rotation between days with low and high carbohydrate intake, while designating both Saturday and Sunday as days with higher carbohydrate consumption. During the low carbohydrate days, it is advised to adhere to a daily limit of 15 net grams of carbohydrates. The calculation of net carbohydrates involves subtracting the dietary fiber consumed throughout the day from the overall quantity of carbohydrates.

Subsequently, one can transition to a conventional routine, dividing meals into lower-calorie or higher-calorie options, with the exception of Sunday which permits indulgence in a treat. For optimal acceleration of weight loss, it is suggested to consider multiplying the ratio of lower carb to higher carb days, potentially up to a doubling or tripling of the current ratio.

When considering the synchronization of carb cycling with your overall schedule, it is crucial to ensure that the days on which you consume the highest amount of carbohydrates align with the days on which you diligently engage in exercise. Given the high-intensity nature of your physical exertion, your body's inherent demand for increased carbohydrate consumption necessitates making immediate and efficient use of an abundance of these energy-providing macronutrients. Please remember to reduce your intake of nutritious fats during days with elevated carbohydrate consumption in order to maintain a harmonious nutritional balance.

Please be aware that the presence of the carbohydrate green light does not grant permission to consume unhealthy carbohydrates. It is advisable to consume complex carbohydrates that provide sustained energy over an extended duration instead. Opt for sweet potatoes, brown rice, and dark, leafy vegetables while actively refraining from consuming high fructose corn syrup by all means necessary. Fructose poses a significantly greater challenge for muscular energy utilization, thereby increasing the likelihood of its eventual storage as fat prior to finding a purpose for it.

Sweet Potato Waffles

Ingredients:

½ teaspoon salt

1 ½ teaspoons vanilla

1 teaspoon cinnamon

2 eggs

½ teaspoon nutmeg

1 sweet potato, cooked and peeled (if desired)

1 cup almond flour

⅓ cup almond milk

2 tablespoons coconut flour

½ tablespoon coconut oil

½ teaspoon baking soda

2 tablespoons maple syrup

Directions:

Combine all of the dry ingredients in a bowl and thoroughly blend them together.

Combine all of the liquid ingredients in a separate bowl, ensuring that the sweet potato is thoroughly mashed.

Integrate the dry and wet components thoroughly by merging them together.

Dispense a portion of the batter onto a preheated waffle iron (sufficient to achieve full coverage) and employ a spatula to smoothly distribute it.

Cook the waffle for an estimated duration of 5 minutes, although it is recommended to closely monitor the cooking process as this timeframe may fluctuate based on the temperature of the waffle iron and the quantity of batter applied.

Principles Of Clean Eating

In each novel dietary program or regimen, there exist underlying principles that form its fundamental basis. These principles serve as the foundation for the entire program or plan. Clean eating can be regarded as more than just a dietary regimen, as it adheres to specific principles. Presented below are several fundamental tenets of maintaining a clean and wholesome dietary regimen.

Eat Whole Foods

Whole foods refer to edibles that exist in their unprocessed, unrefined state. This indicates that they have not undergone any form of processing or alteration within a manufacturing facility or scientific setting. For instance, the inherent state of an apple fruit is achieved when it is plucked directly from the tree. It undergoes processing and modification during the juice extraction process, wherein sweeteners and flavorings are incorporated to create commercially packaged apple juice that is ready for consumption. Contrarily, homemade apple pies, apple marmalades, and apple cider retain their suitability for wholesome consumption as they undergo preparation in personal settings, devoid of factory processing techniques, thereby abstaining from the inclusion of chemical substances and artificial additives. Unprocessed food products are sourced directly from agricultural fields. A few illustrations encompass whole grains, freshly produced fruits and vegetables, unsalted nuts and seeds, among other options.

Avoid Processed Foods

Certainly, it is essential to refrain from consuming processed foods if adhering to a clean eating regimen that solely encompasses all-natural or whole food choices. Processed foods have labels. Upon careful observation of the packaging, it is apparent that the aforementioned food item contains supplementary ingredients, preservatives, and synthetic additives, which contribute to its extended shelf life and uniform taste, comparable to other similar products. Certain food items, such as natural cheeses and whole grain pasta, are subject to processing within factory environments. However, it is important to note that the absence of artificial ingredients typically renders these products permissible, rather than unfavorable. The key is to refrain from purchasing any food product that exceeds five ingredients or contains ingredients with challenging pronunciations.

Abstain from the consumption of refined sugar.

Although the visually pristine appearance of refined white sugar may suggest a higher level of cleanliness compared to brown sugar, it is advisable to refrain from consuming this particular sugar variety due to its prior refinement in a factory. Refined sugar possesses an artificial sweetness that diverges significantly from the innate, organic sweetness of brown sugar. It is advisable to exclude this item from your dietary intake as it primarily contributes to an excess of caloric intake with minimal nutritional value. In order to enhance the flavor of your food and beverages, alternatives such as brown sugar or honey can be utilized.

Integrate Nutritious Proteins, Carbohydrates, and Beneficial Fats

Certain individuals who embark on a dietary regimen tend to err by eliminating a specific food category, be it carbohydrates, protein, or fat, from their established dietary blueprint. This is deemed detrimental to one's well-being as the body necessitates these essential nutrients. You can ensure a well-rounded diet by consuming a nutritionally balanced meal comprising appropriate proportions of protein, carbohydrates, and fats to meet your body's requirements. The integration of these nutrients additionally fosters a heightened sense of contentment and satiety, thereby minimizing the indulgence in unhealthy snacking or excessive consumption. Furthermore, this amalgamation provides an ample amount of sustenance for your body, enabling you to sustain optimal energy levels throughout the entirety of the day.

Prepare your Own Meals

Rather than dining out, it is advisable to contemplate on cooking your own meals within the confines of your home. Additionally, it is advisable to contemplate the option of preparing and bringing your own lunch when commuting to your workplace. This is the optimal course of action if you intend to embark on a clean eating regimen, as it assures that the components employed in meal preparation are entirely derived from nature, and without any processing. It is advisable to refrain from purchasing pre-packaged or instant meals due to their tendency to contain synthetic additives and ingredients. You have the opportunity to experiment with the various recipes that are featured within the contents of this book.

Eat Smaller Meals

Rather than consuming two or three substantial meals throughout the day, it would be beneficial to opt for a dietary pattern consisting of five to six smaller meals. This approach not only enhances your metabolic rate but also ensures a prolonged feeling of satiety, which aids in the prevention of impulsive snacking or binge eating episodes.

Avoid High Calorie Drinks

It is advisable to refrain from consuming high-calorie beverages such as coffee or soft drinks due to their contribution of approximately 400 to 500 calories per day, which can be challenging to expend. Clean eating does not necessitate the meticulous tracking of calorie intake, yet it also does not permit unrestricted consumption of high-calorie foods and beverages at one's discretion. If you are experiencing thirst, you have the option of hydrating yourself with water, unsweetened tea, or freshly squeezed fruit juice.

Balsamic Tomato Bruschetta

Ingredients:

- 2 large garlic cloves minced
- 1 Tablespoons of high quality balsamic vinegar
- 1 teaspoon of olive oil
- ¼ teaspoon of sea or kosher salt
- ¼ teaspoon of black pepper
- 1 loaf of French bread sliced and toasted.
- 8 plum or Roma tomatoes de-seeded and diced
- 1/3 cup of basil chopped
- ¼ of parmesan cheese shredded

Instructions

Incorporate tomatoes, cheese, basil, and garlic into a sizable bowl. Incorporate the balsamic vinegar, olive oil, salt, and pepper. Ensure that the mixture is fully covered and allow it to marinate in the refrigerator for a minimum of 30 minutes, allowing the flavors to amalgamate.

Upon being prepared for serving, place the slices of French bread on a baking sheet and generously drizzle them with olive oil. Transfer the marinated tomato mixture into a serving spoon and proceed to present it.

Creating A Meticulously Crafted Diet Regimen Tailored To Your Personal Needs, One That Remains Resiliently Adhered To Over The Span Of 30 Consecutive Days.

Excessive weight can give rise to myriad challenges for an individual. Individuals who are experiencing excess weight frequently encounter feelings of physical debilitation and lethargy. Individuals who experience weight-related issues also endure a lack of self-assurance and may even experience symptoms of depression.

By identifying an optimal daily dietary regimen and making modifications to your eating patterns, you can effectively eliminate surplus body fat and cultivate heightened self-assurance. Through adhering to a fat-burning diet, one can effectively acquire sufficient energy to undertake their daily tasks.

You will possess an ample amount of strength; you will possess the ability to think with greater clarity and effectiveness. Primarily, by adhering to a daily dietary regimen, you will experience an enhanced sense of self-esteem.

Initially, altering your daily diet might be quite inconvenient. Transitioning from one's accustomed eating habits to adopting a more optimal dietary regimen proves highly challenging. However, it is also quite simple to formulate and/or discover an optimal fat-burning diet that is convenient to adhere to and one that seamlessly aligns with your lifestyle.

When embarking on a daily dietary regimen, it is advisable to commence with a straightforward meal selection. It is not advisable to attempt a complete overhaul of your dietary habits within a short span of one week; doing so may prove challenging for you to adhere to your fat burning nutritional regimen.

Please ensure that you gradually modify your daily dietary intake over a span of at least 30 days. This approach will facilitate your adaptation to the new eating regimen.

In a gradual manner, endeavor to reduce your consumption of food items that contribute to the accumulation of excess body fats, such as meat, crackers, ice cream, cakes, and similar items.

The Significance Of Maintaining Dedication To Your Dietary Regimen

Engaging in a dietary regimen demands a significant amount of resilience and self-control. This is due to the presence of several limitations throughout the duration of the plan. This is the underlying cause behind the lack of success that numerous individuals encounter in relation to the implementation of their dietary plans.

This has caused numerous individuals to apprehend the concept of dieting as they consistently possess the misguided notion that they would not be capable of adhering to the regimen, resulting in the failure of many diet plans prior to their commencement. Numerous individuals fail to comprehend that a nutritious eating regimen does not pertain to deprivation.

This constitutes a primary factor that dissuades numerous individuals from engaging in dieting, as they perceive it as necessitating a complete abstention from the foods they hold dear. They are failing to articulate to themselves that they have the ability to consume foods they enjoy in moderation without completely abstaining.

This is precisely the reason why a considerable number of individuals are resolutely opposed to engaging in dieting, as they frequently conflate this concept with subjecting oneself to a state of starvation.

Individuals must be aware that in order for a dietary regimen they undertake to yield positive outcomes, it is imperative for them to alter their perception of preferred food choices and demonstrate willingness to make concessions with their personal preferences for a designated period of time. Once again, it appears that the message often goes unnoticed: food should not be perceived as our adversary, but rather our inability to properly distribute and consume it is the issue at hand.

Frequently, a significant portion of the population tends to consume incorrect foods rather than the appropriate ones that should be ingested. This is the focal point of the issue.

It is recommended that we consume five portions of vegetables and three portions of fruits daily in order to obtain the appropriate quantity of necessary nutrients. If this condition is not met, we tend to experience a sense of deprivation and endure hunger pangs. If we adhere to the aforementioned portions of fruits and vegetables in our diet, it is improbable that we will experience frequent episodes of hunger.

This suggests that we can indulge in the food we adore, albeit in moderation, as it is imperative to do so. The portion size presents a significant concern as well. We have become accustomed to consuming oversized portions of fries, large cups of soda, and other beverages to the extent that we overlook the concept of proper serving sizes. It is imperative to refrain from succumbing to any such enticements, and instead, only partake in what is essential.

We ought to consistently bear in mind that adhering to a dietary regimen does not involve deprivation. Therefore, it is imperative to derive satisfaction from the entire process and to motivate ourselves in undertaking it.

One must consistently bear in mind the multitude of favorable facets associated with adhering to a dietary regimen and engaging in weight loss endeavors, rather than succumbing to despondency regarding the surplus weight currently being borne.

It is advisable to maintain a favorable perspective and consistently encourage oneself, despite potential delays in the weight loss journey. Continue to affirm to yourself that you will regain your youthful physique.

Nevertheless, adhering to a dietary regimen does not necessitate an absolute cessation of indulging in activities or food items that bring you pleasure. One can indulge in occasional small pleasures within reasonable limits. You are allowed to enjoy occasional treats in moderation. Following this, select an activity of personal significance and enjoyment to effectively expend the additional calories that have been consumed.

By adopting this approach, you will enjoy twice the advantage. The activities in which you have engaged must be pursuits that you anticipate and derive pleasure from. This would aid in the attainment of superior outcomes. In order to achieve success in adhering to a dietary regimen, it is imperative to possess a strong sense of self-assurance and approach the entire process with a positive mindset. If one is unable to avoid indulging, it would be preferable to refrain from indulging, despite any possible desire to do so.

However, if you experience contentment and a positive disposition towards the entire concept of maintaining a healthy lifestyle through dieting and exercise, indulging in occasional small indulgences within reasonable limits can be deemed as an excellent choice.

Five Key Principles to Facilitate Your Transition

1. Make it a point to cook more frequently.

This method represents perhaps the most straightforward approach to embark on your path towards consuming wholesome foods. By engaging in the preparation of meals, you assert complete authority over every aspect, ranging from the selection of ingredients and their freshness, to the methods employed in their preparation, down to the minutest details such as choice of spices or preferred serving style.

2. Read Your Food Labels!

Upon initiating this practice, assuming you have not already done so, you will commence acquiring a comprehension of the constituents that are being ingested through your dietary intake. Although I do not assert that all food labels provide comprehensive and entirely accurate information, it is important to note that legally they are constrained in their ability to deceive consumers (depending on the jurisdiction), making it a promising initial step.

A valuable guideline to follow is to opt for food items that contain five or fewer ingredients, wherein you possess knowledge, recognition, or the ability to pronounce each ingredient.

3. Refrain from Consuming Highly Processed Foods Under Any Circumstances" "Steer Clear of Highly Processed Foods at Every Possible Opportunity" "Exercise Extreme Caution when it comes to Consuming Highly Processed Foods" "Make Every Effort to Avoid Highly Processed Foods without Compromise

Within the realm of industrial food processing, distinct tiers of processing exist. Many of the foods commonly referred to as "health foods" may undergo minimal processing. For instance, similar to the majority of cashews, quinoa or even oatmeal undergoes minimal processing. This does not imply that you should completely avoid these foods, but rather consistently opt for the ones that undergo minimal processing whenever you are given the option.

If you have recently commenced your pursuit of adopting a clean eating lifestyle, I strongly urge taking gradual steps towards this goal and initially concentrating on eliminating the most detrimental items from your diet: refrain from consuming frozen pizzas, avoid indulging in Twinkies, abstain from consuming hot pockets, and steer clear of TV Dinners. Subsequently, it would be advisable for you to enhance your standards by progressively eliminating additional foods that are processed, albeit not to a significant extent, so that the overall quality of your dietary choices continues to improve gradually over time. This course of action is appropriate only if you are able to provide substitute options for the ones you exclude, and if you possess a proficient understanding that the more wholesome and cleaner your diet is, the more refined your ability to enhance flavors naturally should be. This presents an exceptional opportunity for you to experience not only extraordinary new dishes but also exhilarating new flavors. I believe you comprehend the essence of my point...

4. Refrain from consuming any synthetic flavors and sweeteners.

I must emphasize a crucial argument: artificial flavors and sweeteners cannot be classified as authentic sustenance. It is imperative to recognize that we are indeed confronting a mass-produced food item intentionally developed to override the logical faculties of the human brain and solely stimulate the pleasure centers within the brain's reward system. Recreational substances are designed in a comparable manner. It is not surprising that you desire an increasing quantity without comprehending the rationale behind it.

Indeed, this desire for «more» encompasses two distinct aspects:

The psychological aspect: "This product is void of calories, sugars, and contains a low number of calories." I kindly request an increased allocation of (insert your term here) as it is not considered in the current calculation."

Additionally, there is a physiological aspect to consider: it manipulates the body's desire for sugary foods, thereby posing a challenge to resist indulging in them. It is anticipated that over an extended duration, it will contribute to weight gain.

The human body lacks the necessary mechanisms to effectively process synthetic chemicals upon their internalization, thereby presenting a substantial risk to overall well-being.

Although processed foods are primarily associated with the presence of various artificial substances, it is essential to acknowledge that they are not the sole culprits. Beverages, condiments, and seasoning blends also fall within this category, and in certain regions, even everyday items like salt may be subject to artificial chemical augmentation.

5. Watch Your Macronutrient Balance

The macronutrients encompass the components of your diet that consist of carbohydrates, proteins, and fats. These constitute the fundamental components of your dietary intake. I would not encourage excessively fixating on meticulous quantification initially. However, it is highly recommended to develop a fundamental awareness of daily macronutrient intake, particularly during the early stages of embarking upon a nutrition regimen.

It is notable that carbohydrates derived from processed food sources accumulate more rapidly, while simultaneously, there may be an inadequate intake of fats that are beneficial for cardiovascular health.

When you incorporate a diet consisting of predominantly nutritious foods that are abundant in high-quality macronutrients throughout your daily routine, you will experience prolonged satiety, increased energy levels, and optimized bodily functions across various aspects.

May I reiterate: incremental progress is key. Even slight modifications to your macronutrient distribution and gradual adjustments to your dietary patterns in favor of clean eating will yield substantial benefits to both your physique and overall well-being.

The objective here is to establish a properly harmonized system of meals for a majority of occasions by comprehending the genuine repercussions of the dietary selections one makes.

An In-Depth Analysis Of Contemporary Dietary Patterns

In the preceding chapter, we explored the augmented incidence of cancer and other chronic ailments among individuals with inadequate nutritional status. This is particularly evident in cases where processed foods are implicated. Microwave popcorn, compressed fish particles, and high fructose corn syrup, all contain a significant amount of chemical compounds and preservatives. Over half of the typical American diet consists of extensively processed food items, and the advantage of this is that it is quite straightforward to recognize the items we should avoid. Fortuitously, I am here to provide guidance to you, esteemed reader, in facilitating the attainment of this objective and facilitating your comprehension of the underlying principles.

The prosperous corn industry, supported by both subsidies and influential advocates, facilitated the adoption of an inexpensive byproduct, generated through chemical processes, into various commonly consumed food products and beverages. With the aid of an enzyme obtained from the largest bacteria responsible for producing antibiotics and bioactive compounds, High Fructose Corn Syrup was inconspicuously integrated into the contemporary Western diet. Owing to its chemical composition and potent nature, this indulgent additive possesses the capacity to modify our metabolic system, function as an addictive substance, trigger the secretion of adipogenic hormones, suppress our immune system, impair the functioning of the liver and cardiovascular system, foster the development of diabetes and obesity... The catalogue of potential hazards associated with this prominent chemical could extend considerably. Moreover, it pervades all aspects. If you do not typically examine the Nutritional Fact label on your food, it is recommended to start doing so. A considerable quantity of food products, including some unconventional ones, prominently feature high fructose corn syrup (HFCS) as a primary ingredient, often alongside a range of complex components difficult to articulate.

If only the consumption of "preservatives" and "additives" could manifest as the preservation of our youthful vitality and the extension of our mortal existence. One of the primary challenges encountered while navigating contemporary dietary practices lies in comprehending the underlying reasons for the inclusion of certain food items in our meals. While the Federal Drug Administration is believed to have a specific purpose, it is worth noting that they are not immune to unethical behavior and questionable practices within the industry (evidenced by the concept of quid pro quo relationships).

We frequently witness the approval of hazardous substances and the use of the label 'generally recognized as safe' solely for the purpose of maximizing financial gain. The food and agriculture industry is often profoundly swayed by financial considerations, making it challenging for the ordinary individual to distinguish between choices made for personal well-being and those driven by monetary interests. Aspartame, BHA (BUTYLATED HYDROXYANISOLE), Benzene, Monosodium Glutamate, Food Coloring, Xylitol, Splenda - this enumeration continues indefinitely, as these substances are chemical derivatives originating from agriculture or petroleum. All of these substances have demonstrated potential hazards, including leukemia, tumors, and blood cancers, as evidenced by scientific research.

The corporations that exert supremacy in the food and agriculture sector also possess significant interests within the realms of agrochemicals and biotechnology. As we distance ourselves from processed foods, it is crucial to acknowledge additional chemicals that may infiltrate your diet. Over the course of many years, the agricultural sector has grappled with the persistent demand for pesticides and herbicides to protect their crops. Prior generations might

Reflect upon the extensive utilization of DDT and the ensuing controversy arising from its perceived carcinogenic qualities. In the realm of traditional agriculture, various types of pesticides are employed, thus warranting meticulous consideration when it comes to cleansing and handling fresh produce for individuals who opt for non-organic farming methods, which eschew the usage of chemical additives.

The agricultural sector, specifically the meat and poultry industry, is commendable in its own right. Owing to the prevalent trend of deregulation and corporate contributions to political causes, this subject matter often engenders a somber ambiance. Summer backyard barbecues exemplify quintessential American tradition, encompassing the act of grilling and savoring succulent cuts of meat such as steaks, burgers, hot dogs, pork chops, brats, chicken breasts, and racks of ribs. In grocery stores, it can be quite effortless to disregard the apparently flawless arrangement of meat products and remain oblivious to the origins of those animals, the conditions in which they were raised, and their dietary intake prior to slaughter. In recent years, there has been increasing scrutiny towards the excessive utilization of antibiotics within the meat and poultry sector. Within the past decade, agriculture has accounted for more than 80% of the total sales of antibiotics. What is the underlying reason behind such a high level of demand? Difficulties arise when agricultural practices expand to an industrial scale, as the emphasis on business operations shifts towards maximizing product output and profit margins.

For an extended period, there has been a lack of oversight or proper regulation of practices, resulting in livestock relying heavily on large quantities of antibiotics to endure their living conditions, as well as the administration of steroids to either sustain the product until it is ready for harvest or administer growth hormones to boost product output and reduce the duration between infancy and slaughter. It was, and perhaps continues to be, prevalent to witness weeks-old chickens that have reached full growth and are grappling to support the burden of their breasts with their developing legs. In 2015, the FDA established restrictions on the utilization of antibiotics or hormones in poultry, a measure that will require several years for widespread implementation and compliance across all farms. Therefore, if it is necessary for you to consume meat, make a concerted effort to ensure its origins are local and scrutinize the information provided on the labels. When selecting food products, it is advisable to prioritize those labeled as grass fed or wild caught, as opposed to farmed alternatives. Additionally, favor options that undergo minimal processing, are free from growth hormones, and do not contain nitrites or nitrates. These aforementioned characteristics should be taken into consideration. Additionally, protein can be obtained from alternative sources that are both appetizing and nutritious, such as legumes, mushrooms, and quinoa.

To conclude, there is a myriad of things to refrain from engaging with. We have provided a table for your convenience, which lists the items to be avoided in your diet along with their sources.

List of Ingredients, their respective Products, Uses, and Potential Side Effects

High fructose corn syrup, commonly abbreviated as HFCS, is a sweetener derived from corn starch.

Aspartame

Xylitol

Saccharin is widely used as an ingredient in condiments, cereals, prepackaged baked goods, yogurts, jams, gum, candy, and frozen foods. It serves as a sweetener and flavor additive. However, its consumption has been linked to various negative effects, including metabolic disturbance, decreased cognitive functioning, weight gain, chemical dependency, and gastrointestinal distress.

Sodium Nitrite and Sodium Nitrate are commonly found in prepackaged meats such as lunch meats, sausage, hot dogs, and bacon, as well as in meat flavoring. They serve as preservatives and color enhancers for red meats. However, their consumption has been associated with an elevated risk of high blood pressure and a slight increase in the risk of cancer.

Partially hydrogenated oils are known to contain saturated and trans fats. These fats can be found in various sources such as palm oil, lard, margarine, microwave popcorn, and crackers. The process of hydrogenation transforms vegetable oils into a semi-liquid consistency, which is commonly used as a filler, flavor enhancer, and for frying purposes. However, the consumption of these oils has been linked to various health issues including coronary heart disease, obesity, liver dysfunction, cancer, as well as memory problems and behavior disorders.

Derive comfort from the understanding that circumstances are transient. Including bad habits. Occasionally, it can be arduous to acknowledge that our mental and physical faculties are not merely fatigued, but also deprived of nourishment. It is imperative to consistently approach tasks with a composed, assured, and optimistic mindset in order to undertake the required actions for attaining the desired life outcomes. While individuals may prioritize immense wealth and exponential financial success, it is important to note that attaining a superior standard of living and maintaining optimal well-being are key contributors to genuine happiness. Lacking mental and physical fortitude can present significant challenges in the pursuit of one's aspirations and the realization of one's objectives. Now, I shall outline the subsequent procedures...

Exclude the aforementioned foods from your dietary intake. You will be doing a favor to your wallet and physical well-being. Absolutely no inclusion of refined sugars, particularly High Fructose Corn Syrup, as well as the strictly restricted presence of saturated or trans-fats, and processed foods. The primary objective is to prioritize the consumption of food items that have undergone minimal processing, ensuring the shortest possible distance from its source to your plate, while also featuring ingredients known to you. Refrain from the consumption of excessive amounts of sodium and sugar. Avoid wheat.

Adhere to a well-balanced diet with a strong emphasis on the inclusion of vegetables. Vegetables are rich in nutrients, offer pleasurable taste, and boast low caloric content. This particular lifestyle does not impose any limitations on food quantity or caloric intake.

Meat in moderation. If one chooses to consume meat, it is advisable to opt for locally sourced, pasture-raised, or sustainably harvested varieties.

Drink Clean. Water proves to be a beneficial companion. Alcohol is a depressant beverage that contains a significant amount of sugar and constitutes a source of empty calories, therefore it should be consumed in moderate amounts. Fruit juices are widely known for their inherent duplicitous nature. Irrespective of whether your beverage is non-concentrated and you personally witnessed the juicing process of fruits and vegetables into your cup, what you currently hold in your possession is essentially a sweetened liquid. The process of juicing results in the depletion of essential phytonutrients and fiber, which are crucial elements that contribute to the substantial benefits of fruits and vegetables. This leaves you with a product that possesses low digestibility and a propensity for weight gain.

Find your inner Chef. Americans have exhibited a longstanding preoccupation with convenience, often overlooking the potential adverse impacts on their health. Preparing meals for oneself and others is a gratifying and pleasurable endeavor. In the event of feeling apprehensive, commence by utilizing familiar ingredients and gradually explore unfamiliar foods and flavors. In the subsequent chapter, we shall delve deeper into this particular stage.

Mediterranean Tuna Salad

- 2 tablespoons slivered basil leaves
- 3 tablespoons olive oil
- Juice of 1 lemon
- Salt and fresh ground pepper, to taste
- 1 (6-ounce) can or jar of tuna (packed in spring water)
- 1/2 cup artichoke hearts, diced
- 1/2 cup pitted Kalamata olives, chopped
- 1 roasted red pepper, chopped
- 1/4 cup fresh chopped parsley

Incorporate all the ingredients in a bowl and enhance with a suitable amount of salt and pepper. Allow the dish to cool suitably before it is presented.

Present the dish within lettuce leaves, a baguette, or whole grain crackers.

The Association Between Stress And Weight Gain

Surprisingly, there are a multitude of scientifically substantiated mechanisms by which stress can impact and contribute to the weight gain that becomes evident upon stepping onto the weighing scales. The most straightforward of these methods is associated with the stress-induced hormone known as cortisol. A biological aspect of the human physique involves the activation of the 'fight or flight' response, which occurs when the body is subjected to stress. This response prompts the release of specific hormones into the bloodstream, preparing the body to react accordingly.

In its basic and elemental form, the human body lacks the ability to differentiate between the strain incurred from persistent, overwhelming work demands and that arising from situations presenting evident and imminent peril. As a result, regardless of the underlying cause of our stress, the body reacts as if we are on the verge of encountering harm, thereby compelling us to engage in vigorous efforts to ensure our survival or flee swiftly.

The body's response involves triggering surges of energy through the release of adrenaline, redirecting metabolic processes and blood circulation to accommodate intense physical exertion, the secretion of hormones such as cortisol, and several other concomitant physiological alterations. These techniques exhibit notable efficacy in withstanding perilous circumstances; however, should this condition persist for a prolonged duration owing to chronic stress, it may evolve into a legitimate jeopardy to one's well-being. In addition to a plethora of other health complications that may ensue, weight gain is a prevalent consequence of prolonged stress. Hence, certain dietary supplements have been developed to combat the hormone cortisol.

What is the mechanism by which stress and cortisol contribute to weight gain?

Metabolic alterations: It is often observed that individuals experience weight gain while experiencing prolonged periods of stress, notwithstanding the absence of any modifications in their dietary patterns. This phenomenon occurs due to an excessive presence of cortisol in the individual's system, which has the capacity to impede metabolic functioning and increase susceptibility to weight gain beyond their typical propensity. Additionally, this gives rise to heightened challenges when attempting to adhere to a diet regimen with optimal effectiveness.

Cravings: Comfort eating. One may be experiencing the burden of stress, hunger, and be presented with the option of indulging in a nutritious green salad or succumbing to the temptation of a tub of chocolate ice cream. Which is more appealing? When experiencing heightened levels of stress, individuals frequently develop a preference for food items that possess higher fat, sugar, or salt content. These typically include confectionery, processed edibles, and indulgent treats, which are largely recognized as detrimental to one's well-being. These categories of foods are generally more prone to inducing weight gain compared to their healthier alternatives.

Alterations in blood glucose levels: Prolonged stress has the potential to influence an individual's glycemic balance, resulting in emotional instability, exhaustion and somnolence, and occasionally severe complications such as hyperglycemia. Intense stress has also been identified as a potential factor contributing to metabolic syndrome, a composite of health conditions that can eventually escalate into grave complications such as diabetes or cardiac events.

Heightened adipose tissue accumulation: Research findings indicate that excessive and prolonged stressful conditions can significantly influence the distribution of adipose deposits in the body. More precisely, research has demonstrated that increased levels of stress correlate with elevated levels of abdominal fat. Regrettably, adipose tissue accumulated in this specific area not only lacks aesthetic appeal, but also engenders heightened health hazards, including a higher susceptibility to diabetes, compared to adipose tissue stored in alternative body regions.

What are additional pathways by which stress contributes to an increase in body weight?

Emotional eating: Alongside the emergence of cravings for less nutritious food, escalated cortisol levels can contribute to heightened restlessness, prompting increased consumption of food beyond one's customary intake. Individuals who are subjected to stress tend to engage in excessive consumption of palatable foods even in the absence of hunger.

The prevalence of fast food: A commonly acknowledged hypothesis surrounding the escalating rates of obesity in contemporary society is the notion that individuals' demanding lifestyles and excessive workloads impede their ability to dedicate time towards preparing nutritious homemade meals. Given its convenient accessibility, individuals are likely to prefer visiting the nearest drive-thru or placing a takeaway order instead.

Insufficient time for physical activity: Amidst a crowded agenda and urgent responsibilities, one of the initial sacrifices is often the adherence to a regular exercise routine. The majority of individuals do not prioritize their exercise regimen, as contemporary lifestyles have become increasingly sedentary compared to previous generations. Furthermore, our minds are preoccupied with the multitude of stresses and pressures that accompany modern living. Exercise is widely disliked by many individuals, nevertheless, a dearth of physical activity will promptly result in an overall increase in body weight.

If you believe you are experiencing this situation, or if you feel at risk of being overwhelmed by stress, there is no need to worry. There are actions you can take to reverse this pattern of weight gain and simultaneously decrease both your waistline and stress level. These measures include:

• Stress Reduction and Coping Strategies • Managing and Alleviating Stress • Techniques for Effective Stress Management

The primary aspect to prioritize in the pursuit of cortisol reduction involves acquiring the skills to effectively regulate and mitigate stress. Practices such as Tai Chi, yoga, and meditation have the potential to bring about a sense of inner serenity, while employing strategies like maintaining a stress journal can aid in recognizing recurring sources of stress. It is essential to establish boundaries and exercise the ability to decline requests from friends and family when one's commitments become overwhelming. If lacking the necessary time or energy, it is imperative to grant oneself leniency. Additionally, allocating time for activities that bring genuine enjoyment is of equal significance, recognizing that leisure and gratification hold comparable value in the broader context of one's life. Certain stressors may be inevitable, such as the demands and setbacks experienced in the workplace. However, through acknowledging these stressors and discovering strategies to mitigate their impact, individuals can effectively diminish their persistent levels of stress.

• Maintaining a Proper Diet

Cortisol plays a significant role in the regulation of blood glucose levels. By managing your glucose consumption effectively, you can alleviate the strain on your adrenal glands and facilitate a reduction in cortisol levels. Strive to consume three meals per day, complemented by two nutritious snacks interspersed throughout. Refrain from consuming foods that have inflammatory properties, such as those with high levels of saturated and trans fats but insufficient fiber content. Instead, prioritize the consumption of foods that are rich in fiber, specifically those that originate from the ground. It is recommended that men aim for a daily fiber intake of 30-38 grams, while women should target 21-25 grams. Additionally, it is advised to prioritize the consumption of foods that are abundant in omega-3 fatty acids, while minimizing the intake of refined carbohydrates, caffeine, and, whenever feasible, alcohol.

• Appropriate Meal Times

Equally significant to managing the contents of your diet is the matter of meal timing. Throughout the course of consuming food, there is a natural elevation in cortisol levels. Therefore, it is advisable to commence the day with a substantial meal and subsequently reduce its proportion as the day unfolds. Consume your breakfast within one hour of arising and ensure a maximum interval of 4 hours between subsequent meals.

• Please commence your journey promptly.

Aerobic or cardiovascular exercise can exert a direct impact on diminishing cortisol levels within the body, while simultaneously accelerating the metabolism to facilitate the elimination of surplus calories responsible for weight gain. Although there is undoubtedly truth in the notion that exercise contributes to stress reduction and cortisol regulation, it is essential to acknowledge that excessive physical activity can actually have a counterproductive effect, placing significant strain on the adrenal glands. It is advisable for individuals experiencing stress and who have relatively low fitness levels to utilize a heart rate monitor and ensure that their heart rate remains below 90 beats per minute during the engagement in anaerobic exercise. This can be gradually introduced by initiating a brisk walk lasting 15-20 minutes, progressively transitioning to light jogging as your physical condition improves. Please proceed with the task, but exercise caution to avoid excessive efforts or overexertion.